Miracle or Mental Illness:

You've Asked the Question

by

Shelley J. Madkins

DORRANCE
PUBLISHING CO
EST. 1920
PITTSBURGH, PENNSYLVANIA 15238

All quotes for technical information are as per Debbie Griffin, Rn, Psychology and Mental health nurse.

Dorrance Publishing Co
585 Alpha Drive
Pittsburgh, PA 15238
Visit our website at *www.dorrancebookstore.com*

ISBN: 978-1-4809-3832-8
eISBN: 978-1-4809-3855-7

This book is dedicated to the loving memory of my mother, Thelma P. Madkins. Rest in peace butterfly rest.

This book is also dedicated to anyone that has a dream.

"Dreamer"
If it's real to your heart,
make it real to your being,
the first path of a dream,
lies in your forseeing.

So if you believe it, it will come true!
Set your dreams high,
Persist and pursue!

By Shelley J. Madkins

For the longest time I have contemplated writing my story. My only apprehensions lie in the repercussions I could perceivably encounter. Was I ready to say to some that I, for a time, had belonged in the unjust niche they had so readily placed me? Was I ready to say, "Demon I know your wicked ways" and "I know how to diminish your voices when you magnify them so." When I determined that I could possibly help someone whose loved one is in a state of utter disillusion, yes even in their darkest hour, I decided to write on. Not only do I feel I can help someone, but it affords me the opportunity to lay this demon to rest. Medication and counseling can also help, and does help. Yet it does not eradicate it completely. This demon was so strong that I tried to kill myself several times. Now, you are probably wondering what this demon is and why kill yourself over an inner-demon. Well, the demon that I speak of is called schizophrenia. Schizophrenia is a "biological illness that involves chemical imbalances in the brain called neurotransmitters." "Two of these neurotransmitters are dopamine and serotonin." "Neurotransmitters carry messages within the brain." In simpler terms, schizophrenia affects the brain which makes it a mental illness.

Society sometimes says that anybody affected with any type of mental illness is to be medicated and locked away from so-called normal society. Well, today I take a stand, compelled to paint a picture that is as vivid as the color red, to take you to another dimension, the world of schizophrenia.

"Schizophrenia is not genetic, but there is a susceptibility to getting the illness that runs in families." I must state that no one in my family has schizophrenia, just me.

I also chose to write about the struggles of schizophrenia to give another perspective of the schizophrenic. I want to crush the ideology that all schizophrenics are disgruntled, white, middle aged men who kill. This has been perpetuated very often in the media. Schizophrenia has been around forever. However, I can probably count on one hand the number of women with schizophrenia, or any other mental illness, that go out into the community and kill. I recall Andrea Yates, the white female who killed all of her children, but not many others. You are bound to get more schizophrenic women who comply with their treatment plans than men. Men think if they feel good one day, then they do not need their medicines that day. Doing this sets them right up for a relapse, which sometimes means a trip to a mental health facility.

Read on in my book and see how I discovered that schizophrenia is not a white man's disease at all.

Schizophrenia manifests itself differently in each person it affects. The big problem that I had during my first bout was the inability to decipher between reality and nonreality. Some of the general symptoms of schizophrenia I will expand upon. However, how it affected me personally, I will get to that part of my story later.

"Distortions in perceptions and thinking that are found in people with schizophrenia is called 'Positives'." "They are called positives because they are added to everyday experiences, not because they are good." "Examples of hallucinations are smelling, feeling, tasting, hearing things that only the schizophrenic experiences." "Some examples are paranoid delusions: people believe they are going to be harmed, or are in danger." Schizophrenics believe and are in constant fear and anxiety. "Referential delusions: an example is thinking and knowing that the male or female on the television is sending special messages." "Somatic delusions: is the idea that something is wrong with their bodies." Auditory hallucinations are hearing voices or sounds that other people do not hear. Persecutory hallucinations are when the voices attack you personally. Often these hallucinations are mean and insulting. Visual hallucinations are seeing things others do not see. "They can be nonspecific or flashes of images." These can also be brought on by visual prone drugs like LSD or marijuana. "Tactile hallucinations are sensations of something on the skin." "Olfactory hallucinations: are sensations of unpleasant odors."

Now that we have gone over the different types of hallucinations, we can get to the meat of my schizophrenia, and the symptoms that I suffered. So, when does schizophrenia begin? The first symptoms of schizophrenia usually appear between the late teens and the mid-thirties. However, sometimes it is later, because I have a friend who didn't get it until the mid-forties, which is sometimes much later. "Most of the time symptoms develop gradually with the earliest signs of the illness appearing years before the psychotic symptoms actually show up." "Early signs include becoming more and more isolated from friends and family, having poor sleep habits, acting like a totally different person doing poorly in school."

So now you are probably wondering how schizophrenia is diagnosed. "There is currently no blood test or any other medical test to make a diagnosis." "It cannot be diagnosed on a single incident or symptom." "Rather, the diagnosis is based on a pattern of sign and symptoms that are present." "A doctor conducts a careful interview and performs a physical exam." "There also may be signs that other people have observed."

"Another set of symptoms are negative and cognitive symptoms." "Negative symptoms take away a person's interest, motivations, and abilities." "Another negative symptom is when the schizophrenic does not show feelings and has a flat affect," pretty much emotionless. "The schizophrenic does not feel like doing anything and could like staying in bed all day." "Schizophrenics feel no pleasure (well sort of), are not interested in having fun and sometimes have no social interests." "Cognitive symptoms include problems with concentration, attention, and learning." "Cognitive is a medical word for thinking. This does not mean a low I.Q." "Trouble planning and thinking things through which make it harder to learn new skills." I consider myself to be relatively intelligent, so when it came to the reality or nonreality method of deciphering what was going on, my intellect made it much harder for me. Hence, my inability to decide what was going on made me more afraid.

Now, I'd like to try and explain how schizophrenia is treated. Schizophrenia is treated using antipsychotic medications. "People with schizophrenia almost always need medication to control and semi-live with their symptoms." "The word antipsychotic means something that blocks or stop psychotic symptoms. They affect the brain chemicals that are imbalanced. Some antipsychotic medications are Haldol and Loxapine. Loxapine is the generic of Loxatane. The treatment of antidepressants are also used to put the chemical imbalances back in balance. Schizophrenics and family of schizophrenics should not get discouraged or give up if the first medication or medications does not work, there are many that may help. "Keep the faith!"

"Conventional antipsychotics have been around for a long time." "They help by blocking some affects of dopamine in the brain."

"Along with the conventional antipsychotics, there are atypical antipsychotics." "Atypical antipsychotics or newer medications that work on two different chemical messengers in the brain, dopamine and serotonin." "They may also help with negative symptoms." "They have less side effects which could include feeling tired, stiffness in arms or legs, hand tremors, tongue movements, and weight gain. Many of the side effects can be managed by the doctor, so again, do not give up, and family and friends you can be the beacon of hope that keeps the schizophrenic from falling further and further out of reality. The further out of reality that the schizophrenic gets, and how we compensate for the voices and why we are hearing them, the harder it is to get back into reality.

The best way that I can explain what schizophrenia is like is when you walk into a haunted house at a theme park. You don't know what to expect. You go through bumps, twists and turns that scare you into oblivion. You see things and hear things that nobody else hears or sees. Another example of what schizophrenia is like is that it is eternal damnation. If schizophrenia is in any way indicative of what hell is like, then I don't want to go there, and neither do you. I feel that I have a call on my life to save schizophrenics and to enlighten all as to what hell could possibly be like.

In the bible it states that hell is going to be a place where there is eternal torture. Imagine, until eternity, that means forever! I'm sure that we all can understand the lake of fire. If you are a Christian and God is in your life regularly, then the majority of your hallucinations and delusions will be on the religious side; at least mine were. Not only did I have delusions and hallucinations, but I had what we call in the psychiatric world "thought-broadcast." Thought-broadcast is when your thoughts are heard through the radio, television, in-person and through buildings and walls connected to wherever you are. If I am nowhere near radio, or television, then these mediums would not harm me, just the people in my vicinity and again that is in-person and through buildings.

I know you are probably thinking she is delusional now as she writes. Some people admit to hearing me, while others do not. That is why I am the quintessential schizophrenic. I actually hear comments from the radio, TV and people around me. This can be in some ways uncomfortable because, just like you are hearing me, well, I in return can hear you. If you are thinking to yourself, then it won't go in my ear! However, unlike you, I do not hear or see things you are privately thinking, only if you talk it out. You know, within my past twenty years I have often asked whether what I am experiencing is a miracle or mental illness. I know that I have schizophrenia, but did God put this on me, or is my imbalance just that strong? Well, as I speak to you via my writings, I am sure that God put this on me because only God can make this happen. I just need to know if this is a result of schizophrenia.

Most doctors in the psychiatric field have heard of thought-broadcast but do not know how to treat it, just with an older antipsychotic and sometimes more than one antipsychotic. I am treating my schizophrenia with Haldol, Loxapine and Seroquel, all of which are antipsychotics. I am also treating my illness with an antidepressant called Citalopram. I take a pill called Benztropine. This is a generic pill of Cogentine used to prevent many of the side effects associated with psychiatric medicines.

Now I know that you are probably wondering when did I get sick and how did it manifest itself in my life. Let me first say that nothing scared me except God, but when I first got sick I thought of everything that was happening that I now was afraid of, and they were all internal, my hallucinations that is.

In April of 1988, when I awoke everything was different. The birds chirped louder. There was an eerie silence like I never heard before, and I was afraid! I had not slept well and I was sweating. I called out to my momma, "Momma! Momma!"

She responded, "Why won't you come down here?"

I just continued to call her, "Momma!" "Momma!"

She came upstairs and asked me, "Why are you crying?" I just kept on crying. She left and went downstairs. Then my brother came upstairs and was trying to see what was wrong with me. When he left and went downstairs, I put together some money and pictures of my nephew and niece. I jumped out of a two story window and planned on going to the church I grew up going to, but it was locked. I thought they were trying to kill me so I got on a bus trying to get as far away from home as possible. Every time I ended up going somewhere that was familiar to me. I saw a lot of people I knew, or thought I knew, and would take off running in the opposite direction. I heard trucks backfire and thought that someone was shooting at me.

The driver said, "Do you think that somebody is shooting at you?" I just kept running. I ran out into traffic trying to get hit several times on this day. I was at another bus stop and my brother saw me, because he had been looking for me. He got out of his car and put me in his car.

He asked me, "Where are you going?"

I cried out, "They are trying to kill me! They are trying to poison me!" He just laughed and took me home. When I returned home my eyes were bloodshot red from jumping out the second story window. Then, around 9:30 P.M. this same day, my momma got off from work. She and my brother took me to the hospital where she worked and the doctor found nothing wrong with me. This was the beginning of my schizophrenia. Some say that we are born with schizophrenia and between our late teenage years and mid-thirties is when it would manifest itself. I was twenty-five, two months away from twenty-six.

After I got home from the hospital I went upstairs and took my bible and read it out loud all night long, reading wherever I opened that bible. I read and experienced the first hallucination of my life. I had not slept, and it was early Saturday morning and I heard a lot of people outside of my brother's window. When I went to look out of his window, all I saw was a little dog walking down the street. I then turned to ask my brother if he had heard anything and he said "no." I then was looking at cartoons on TV and I heard it say, "Lucifer is dead, Lucifer is dead." Again, I heard "Lucifer is dead, Lucifer is dead." I heard and checked my pulse to reassure myself they were not talking about me. I could not have then explained why I heard a lot of people outside my brother's window. I did not know why or how I heard a lot of people. I also did not know that I was hallucinating. The very next day I was looking at the TV and I was receiving messages from the TV. Exactly what, I don't recall, but I guess this was my first experience with the thought-broadcasting. This time it was substantially different; people around me could not hear me and people outside could not hear me. The only people that could hear me were the people on TV and the people on the radio. This was in the year of 1988.

Between the month of April 1988 until February of 1989 I was not sleeping, just resting my eyes. The unbelievable hallucinations that followed were deep. As I mentioned earlier about some of the hallucinations, the ones that manifested in my deepest, darkest time were the persecutory hallucinations and the auditory hallucinations.

Many of the persecutory hallucinations were sexual in nature. The persecutory and the auditory hallucinations worked hand-in-hand. Every night I would get raped and stabbed, however, the odd thing about this was that the hallucinations that were raping me took on the personality of men and women whom I was familiar with. I couldn't imagine how they could do this. The hallucinations continued all night long. I did not sleep at all. I actually felt movement in my vagina, butt and mouth. The hallucinations took turns and I was sick, just as if it had happened for real. When the voices stabbed me it really hurt. The voices were saying, "Die bitch, die bitch." I remembered that my spirit was trying to come out of my body. I would feel it lifting up and when I breathed in then my spirit would come back into my body. Again, the voices would say "die bitch, die bitch."

Guess what my logic was for this? In my intellectual mindset, it was that all people except for me could turn themselves into ghosts and do this to me. The voices would hit me over the head with bats and sticks. I remember playing dead several times, but my spirit would always come back into my body. When I breathed in, this would happen again and again, all night long for about seven months. I even resolved it within myself that my momma's house was haunted.

Every morning I would get out of bed and sit with my momma while she drank her coffee. She would ask me if I slept and my response was always, "no." She looked very worried. A month later my brothers and sisters became a part of my hallucinations by egging on the men in my hallucinations. I was lost and devastated. I was the walking wounded. Can you imagine that all you know is no longer true!

I remember preparing to go to sleep, I would place my bible on my chest and in between my legs, but I still felt the stabbings and raping. One night I was going to hurt the hallucinations by stabbing in the air. The beating hurt even more. I told my momma I was afraid so she called my sister and they took me to Malcolm Bliss, which is a mental health facility in St. Louis, MO. I was pulling out my hair and I was quite delusional. The voices kept repeating, "We are going to get her, we are going to get her." I was worried that the voices said they were going to get my mother. I didn't tell the intake doctor or nurse that I was afraid for my mother. They admitted me to the mental health facility and I was still afraid. I just could not handle being around all those people so I stayed in my room. I didn't tell them much about the thought-broadcasting, because I thought they could hear me. However, they couldn't at this time in my experience.

The only time that I got some sleep was when I was in the hospital. The short period I was in the hospital I still heard voices and felt sensations. It was at Malcolm Bliss Mental Health Facility that I got my first diagnosis, major depression with psychosis. The only reason that I got this diagnosis was because I lied about myself thinking that someone was trying to kill me or hurt me. As I mentioned earlier in this book, I was not afraid of anything or anybody except God. Yet, the paranoid delusions were in my mind that someone was trying to kill me. Schizophrenia was a continual diagnosis since I thought that people could change themselves into ghosts at night. I wondered what was it that I was not doing that made me unable to do this.

See, what I am saying is I could not have known the difference between reality and nonreality. I was not healing, which happens when we sleep.

My weight this far was 125lbs, but since I was not eating much and not sleeping much, I weighed only 105lbs. My whole world was turned upside down. The world as I knew it was no longer so. I could not give a good explanation of why the devil was attacking me. Maybe it was because I loved Jesus our God so much!

The hallucinating part of schizophrenia is one of the main factors in diagnosing schizophrenia. I could have said that there were ghosts threatening my momma. Had I done this, the diagnosis would have immediately been schizophrenia.

Can you imagine being stabbed and beaten, where the pain is real as it feels? Let me also say that the sexual sensations were not pleasant at all. So don't think that I enjoyed it; it hurt and it was humbling. Just like there would be an odor if a lot of people had sex with me, the odor on me was doubly disgusting.

During my first hospitalization they told me that it would take approximately three weeks until I could be released. I remember the first time I walked on my floor, I looked for a window to jump out. I did this to put myself out of my misery. Meaning if I were to have my back against the wall, I'd have an out! Malcolm Bliss had a lot of floors, and the floor I was on swayed back and forth. I didn't know if that was another hallucination, or not. The hallucinations I had in the hospital were the same as I mentioned earlier plus gun shots being heard, and gun shots being fired into my head. My head felt like an empty hollow shell. When I awoke this particular time I awoke to find one of the aids standing over me!

I remember the following day which was my fifth day, looking at the clock and seeing that it was 6:00. I didn't know if it was A.M. or P.M. so I called home and my niece reassured me that it was A.M. and I had a meeting with the Mental Health Board to determine if I was ready to be released. I lied and told them that I was no longer having symptoms so they released me. I gave some of the board members an evil eye so they said, "If she wants to leave, let her leave. We cannot make her stay if she has surpassed her involuntary status."

My momma, my brother, my niece and my nephew picked me up at 7:00 that evening. The doctor informed my momma not to let me spend the majority of my time alone. I came in and went right upstairs, again being alone. My hallucinations this time were while I sat on the couch in the hall. I had no TV, no stereo, or radio on. I heard five little kids laughing and running into the paneled wall we had upstairs.

Now, you are probably wondering why am I telling you all about these different hallucinations. It is because at the beginning of this book I promised to take you all deep into the darkness of schizophrenia. So get on board. It gets better, or worse; it depends on who you ask. If you ask me, it gets worse. Just imagine that you had never hallucinated before. Wouldn't you think that the place you hallucinated in was haunted? I am sure the devil had something to do with what I was going through. However, why did God allow this to happen? Maybe God let this happen to me because he knew I would tell this story, especially if it is a calling on my life to save the schizophrenic, and to let it be known what hell will be like.

Another time after I went upstairs and I closed my eyes it felt like I was combusting after another hallucination. I was covered with gasoline and I was melting. When I went downstairs to look at myself I saw a burned face and I smelled like fire.

After my short stint in the hospital I was referred to an outpatient clinic called Metro. Here I saw a psychiatrist by the name of Dr. Sadowski. I told her that I could be heard by people in the radio and on television. She quickly told me that this was not possible. She wrote me a prescription for Loxapine and sent me on my way. Maybe this was God's way of preparing me for my new life because seven years later I had the thought-broadcast return. Yet, when it returned, it was completely devastating. I will touch on the second bout with the thought-broadcast later. I thought that Metro was a place where people went to get shots and die. When I was with the therapist she just kept on saying, "And then you'll get your shot."

So I calmed all the way down and said, "I'm ready." I was tired of running and being tortured.

After that she said, "Stop and make an appointment with me in two weeks." My brother and I left and went home.

When my brother and I returned to my mother and father's home he told me to sit in the yard with him and my nephew while he cut the grass. I guess he was trying not to let me isolate. I was sitting in the yard and I started to hallucinate.

I thought that I was pregnant from the sexual sensations that had been happening. I sat there and I was feeling like I was pregnant because when I breathed in there was no sound, but when I exhaled I heard a demonic voice calling me a bitch until it was almost out of the birth canal. Then when I inhaled it came back in, and again with bitch after I exhaled. This went on for about an hour and a half. While this was happening my nephew was saying, "There goes a blue one, there goes a green one, there goes a red one," and so on and so forth. Why was my nephew seeing things that I could not see?

I got up and went inside the house. I hope that I have taken you deep into the darkness of schizophrenia. I am not done but I hope that you all have decided that you would rather go to heaven and stay as far away from hell as possible. Just because I don't mention the sexual sensations does not mean that they stopped. The beatings and the sexual sensations did not end thus far. I was just as disoriented as ever. The other hallucinations were in addition to what was going on at night. This one particular hallucination was that my neck was tied to a car and I was bouncing back and forth in bed, yet the bed rocked and so did I.

Every time I got out of bed, I would take my bible with me. I opened the bible this one time and it said that a Christian should be dressed in white or something to that effect. I took a shower and washed my white short set. I put it on and went to and looked out our front door and I saw a refuse truck pass by. I thought it said for me to refuse sexual advances and so I fought the sexual sensations and was beaten harder and harder.

The medicine that I am on is Loxapine an antipsychotic. I was growing deeper, and deeper into depression and psychosis so I decided to end my life as I knew it. I had this medicine plus some Benadryl. I had gotten quite upset and more and more disoriented so I decided I wanted out. I put a bottle of aspirin, the remaining Loxapine and the remaining Benadryl in a tall cup with water. It was about sixteen ounces of water and medication. I drank it and then I was very afraid so I went into the basement and threw it up. I drank more and more water and then threw it up. I did this time and time again. While I was in the basement I walked around trying not to fall asleep.

My momma came downstairs and looked me in the eye, as if to say, "Tell me it isn't so." She went back upstairs and I continued to walk around the basement. I finally got too tired to walk and fell asleep. I lay down to die. I had a bad dream and I woke up. I said, "This is good," and then I remembered what was going on in my life. I checked my pulse and felt nothing. I went upstairs and told my momma that I was dead. My momma assured me that dead people didn't walk around. She told me to get some greens that she had cooked. Everything inside was dried up and the greens came out of my body just like they were when I put them in. The greens came out undigested; this scared me but, after that my body returned to being moist. Before my body turned back to the way it normally was, the medicine was still in my system.

My momma brought me home a urine cup to fill up. I peed in the cup and there were little white specks floating around in the cup. The doctor set me up a doctor's appointment and I went the following Wednesday. I was going to get a catheter so that the urine would come out. I thought that my momma was taking me to get an abortion. The doctor told me that it was going to hurt. It did not hurt because I was still numb from the Loxapine, Benadryl and aspirin.

I hope that I have given you all insight into schizophrenia. I am sure that this insight is very informative. However, I am not done telling my story.

There are more hallucinations. With my story so far you can see what it is like when a schizophrenic does not take his or her medication as prescribed. Every setback takes him or her deeper into psychosis. Before I get back into the hallucinations, I will tell you what to do after you have found a cocktail of medication that keeps you functional and somewhat stable. Know that you will never be cured from schizophrenia because there is no cure. You just have to tweak your medications until you are functional. There are ways to prevent a relapse. The sooner you get help, the less horrific your journey will be.

So the main way to prevent a relapse is to stay on your medication. It is rare to relapse if you are on your medication. You need to work with your treatment team and keep them informed as to your symptoms. The second best way is you must keep your appointments. It is never a good idea to stop taking your medicine and wait for the next appointment! It is also a good idea to learn as much as possible about schizophrenia. Once you begin to recover from the severe psychotic symptoms of the illness then you are better able to learn more about schizophrenia, how to deal with it and how to prevent a relapse. That is why I wrote this book, so you, as a caregiver, and you as a well schizophrenic, will know the symptoms to look for and you also will know what questions to ask. Such as "Do you think that people are trying to harm you?" "Are you feeling anything different that you don't know what or why it is?" Something to that effect will give you insight as to what is happening in his or her mind. It is very important that you reduce your stress. "Try living with someone you know or with a family member." Then you can get an idea of what you can handle and what you can't handle. You cannot take a full load of classes and work. This is stressful for the normal minded person, let alone the person with a chemical imbalance in the brain. Most of all take your medication every day and how it is prescribed. "Eat a healthy diet, and ask for help when needed." People with schizophrenia are very sensitive to stress so again, ask for help. "People with schizophrenia often need help learning how to hold a job, manage their money, and deal with other aspects of daily living." The treatment team can make it easier to get a schizophrenic's life back on track. The schizophrenic must commit to working with the treatment team and to tell them the truth about what is happening to him or her. "There are several warning signs of relapse: 1) trouble sleeping 2) feeling anxious 3) problems thinking clearly 4) losing interest in people or activities 5) isolating 6) feeling irritable 7) feeling physically ill from lack or withdrawal from not taking prescribed medicine." Family members remember these symptoms and any other symptoms that you can remember from the last relapse. So now you know what to do after you have weighed their responses. If anything is out of the norm get help immediately! Especially if it is a male. Once this book is out, there is no need to let it fester, so get help immediately!

Now back to the hallucinations. My brother, my niece, my nephew and I went to the zoo. As we were leaving to get into the car I heard something that sounded like a gun shot. I hallucinated that something hit my foot. This was where there was an old sore on my foot, so I was limping as if I had been shot. When we got to the zoo at this time, I experienced bad vibes. I was hallucinating when I heard, "You threw my baby off a bridge." I was devastated. Could I actually do something that was so demonic? No, was the answer. Yet, I still felt bad. The voices kept saying things to this effect. I didn't know why since I had taken good care of my niece and nephew.

My most odd hallucination was when I went to sit in the living room one night. I was trying to go somewhere different other than my bedroom thinking this would stop the raping and beatings. Instead I heard the trumpets as the book of revelations warned us about in the last days. I heard the ceiling rolling apart, and then the angels started to sing. I got up and went into my momma's bedroom door and told her that it was over and she shook her head and agreed. She didn't know what I was talking about, she just knew that my life would probably never be the same, and she felt bad for me. As a matter of fact all my friends and family felt sorry for me.

About five months prior I had just completed a bookkeeping/accounting program, and was ready to go back to work. However, the beating about the head made it hard for me to remember what I had studied. Schizophrenia is probably the reason why I really could not remember any of the bookkeeping/accounting. Later in my life it came back to me. I did nothing for about two to three more months. I cleaned house and listened to my voices. I remembered being lonely and I would listen for my voices. The only reason I listened to these voices was because they were religious in nature, and they were safe.

One day my cousin called looking for my momma and she said, "Try the temporary services." I thought, *how can I work when I am being attacked*? I was taking my medicine as it was prescribed. It made me sleepy, but I still could not sleep. So anyway I called a temporary service and made an appointment for two days later. I called a downtown temporary service because I knew my way around downtown. I had a mantra that kept me functioning. That was, "Act like everybody else." After my interview they gave me a position with Pet Incorporated. I was very quiet. After completing this assignment I registered with two other temporary services, and then after that one more. Any time one didn't have an assignment I called a second one and then a third one. I never smiled and my effect was flat. However, I got the assignment finished and correctly finished. The reason I had not been hired at this time was because they said that I was too soft-spoken.

I was convinced that my thought-broadcast this time was just through the radio and TV. So I was never around the radio or the TV. One evening I stood in my momma and dad's room and the TV looked different; they did not respond to my comments and there was a glaze over the TV. Great! My thoughts were no longer going through the radio or TV!

Remember that I stated earlier that the less stress you have as a schizophrenic the better off you will be. Well, during my two years working for thirty-two companies through the temporary services I was sexually harassed a lot. I was not eating right and I didn't like how my medicine made me feel so I quit taking them. I thought that I would never hallucinate again. I thought that I had beaten schizophrenia. Little did I know, I was headed for a relapse. Any time I didn't eat, sleep, or take my medicine, I was headed for a relapse. I was working for this insurance company and this black lady, this black man, this white girl, and this white man who was the boss kept sexually harassing me. So one day I got up and walked away from this job. They were getting on my last nerve. When I got home I started hallucinating again. I heard the voices saying, "They are going to kill your mother. They are going to kill you mother." I got some clothes, my briefcase and some money and took off going to my God mother's house. She was not home so I got on the bus and got to Barnes Jewish hospital. I am not sure if it was Barnes Jewish yet, but I do remember walking down to Jewish hospital and calling my momma and she had me call my sister. She came and got me and took me home. I took some of my medicine and felt better in a day or two. I made an appointment with Metro, the outpatient clinic. I told her that I had been hearing voices. She wrote me a prescription and my brother picked it up. This was where I got the diagnosis of a schizophrenic. I told her everything that I was going through. So, when I first came there I had the right diagnosis.

Paranoid Schizophrenia, which I thought was a white man's disease, is what I have. However, I saw that there are just as many African Americans with schizophrenia. So now I know that it is not just a white man's disease.

After my later episode with hallucinations, I went onto my final assignment this time, with the temporary services. That was the American Red Cross. I worked in the donor updating center. They wanted me to stay there but instead I chose to go to work for the City of St. Louis in the housing courts as a supervisor of the clerical staff. I stayed there for two years until I was racially discriminated against and fired for alleged poor performance. I sued in the federal courts for not complying with the ADA guidelines and the Title VII. We settled out of court for a humble amount because I knew that the City of St. Louis did not have much money. A year and three months after I was fired I moved back home with my parents. I was very distraught about losing my beautiful apartment and over losing my job. I isolated upstairs with my niece and nephew. Guess what came back in September (labor day) in 1995. Right, the thought-broadcasting came back and this time it was stronger. Again, I was so distraught that the only way that I could accept it was by saying, "If it gets worse I'll just kill myself." For years I held on to suicide to make me feel better. "Why had this happened to me again?" Not only could the radio and the TV hear me, but people around me could hear me as well as people outside of whatever buildings, houses, or apartment that I am in. People looked at me differently, and treated me differently. Some called me a witch, while others called me the second messiah. I'll get to the second messiah thing a little bit later.

I remember one of the worst hallucinations I had and that was everybody was at my burning, and that was that I was a witch. I was placed upon a stake and was to be burned. I called out as many names as possible. When I called out their names the familiarity of their voices shocked me and after I called the names they all answered "yes." After this I was doused, my body reeked of fire. I smelled like burning flesh.

My second bout with thought-broadcasting I was instantly suicide prone. My family and friends were dumbfounded. They just could not believe that this had happened to me. I know that they were praying for me because I heard through my thought-broadcasting, "She still has it." I had it again, but contrary to what they heard, this was not the first time that this had happened. When I told them that the radio and the television could hear me back in 1988, they said, "Who do you think you are?" This time they knew I was able to do this because they heard it too. I was still at my parents' house when this happened. I took my TV, a boom box and some CDs and moved into the walk-in closet away from the windows and away from my family. The first thing that I did was put my radio on the gospel station to see if this and prayer would take it away. I started sending and donating money to ministries and ordering tapes and listening to them. I wrote to Joyce Meyers, Dr. Laura Slessinger and an African American Bishop and his wife. I wanted all of them to pray for me. I listened to gospel music; anything that was God and Jesus, I listened to. Even though I listened to radio and TV a lot less, I did make friends with some of the DJs and made friends with one or two of the news reporters on Univision. So, that was how I initially handled the thought-broadcasting. I noticed then and I knew now how irate some of their TV personnel and DJs got when I was just listening to their show without interacting with them per se. Another thing I have with the thought-broadcasting is if I wanted someone to feel something from me, like a tap on the shoulder, then you would feel it, just as if I was in the same room. It is mind-boggling. This is true, I kid you not! When I do this through my thought-broadcasting I hear a response of, "I'm going to church." This is a perfect response because God wants us back in church. So, if I can assist him in doing so, I have appeased him.

However, turnaround is fair play, since I can touch you all, then you all can do the same thing to me. If I, through my thought-broadcasting, wanted to perform a sexual act on whoever is in my vicinity I could do. I won't expound anymore about this right now. A lot of people asked, "How come you hear us?"

My response was "Because you hear me."

I was thirty-three when my thought-broadcasting returned. This time I knew that people could not turn themselves into ghost and attack me sexually. However, when it came back I knew that people outside of my parents' house could do things to me. I responded by sticking them in the eye or something like that. I opted not to do anything sexual because I hated what I was feeling and this might encourage them, no matter who it was. What people can do with their minds felt like I was itching, not physically like in

1988. In 1988 it felt penetrating like it was actual sexual intercourse. I did not enjoy any of it. Maybe I suffered the hallucinations because this was how my new life would be. Maybe I am stuck with the thought-broadcasting or maybe God will change my ability to think without the thought-broadcasting after I tell my story.

Hopefully people who think about sex a lot will change their ways with the fear it may happen to them. Before this and after this I thought about sex a lot. The news reporter that I befriended I thought about sexually even though I am not a lesbian, and neither was she. It was something new, so I dabbled and did things sexually to her. This went on for about three months. After about three months, I received my settlement from the City of St. Louis and I moved out of my parents' home to an upscale apartment complex. I thought this place would be the perfect place and that these people would be too busy to listen to me. However with this place being on a busy intersection, it was just too busy for me. Another reason why I chose this apartment was because I felt it would be nice for the news reporter. I also remembered that we had an understanding that if she was not on the cable system there, then we would just let it go. She was not on their cable so I let it go.

Since this place was so busy, I moved to another apartment in Rock Hill, MO. It was beautifully built and appeared to be quiet. Little did I know that this was going to be one of the worst places that I lived because of a nuisance neighbor. He rung my doorbell constantly. When I got to my door, he would run down to the garage. This happened from day one, ring and run just like a juvenile of some sort. To get away from him I would pack my suitcase and go and stay at a hotel for a couple of days. I know he did this because of the thought-broadcast. Something different about this thought-broadcast is that when I am sleeping or I am falling asleep you cannot hear me. This gave him great joy and as I nodded off he would step or make a noise on the ceiling. There was no reason he did this except he was a racist busybody. He thought that my life was one that could be played with. I was very paranoid, not paranoid scared, just paranoid because there was not enough medicine in my system. So, I was paranoid because I didn't have enough medicine left over. During this time I was just taking one Loxapine a night. This was by no means enough medicine. Sometimes I would go to the pharmacy and get three to four pills and try to make it last for about six to ten days. I did this by opening the capsule and emptying the contents in the vile and I would put some of it on my tongue. This didn't help that much but it's what I did. With people in the connecting apartments making things go through my mind, I was miserable.

Another part of the thought-broadcast that brought me much stress was when a celebrity would die and they put it on the TV live. So, I was very unnerved when Princess Diana died. I knew her funeral would be on TV and I really panicked. I did not want my thoughts to be broadcasted during her funeral so I packed up some clothes and went to a hotel. The way that I knew my thoughts would go through to the TV was because if I am in a building with others, and they have on their TV, then my thoughts go through to the TV station. I just didn't want my thoughts to go through to her service. It did, and I lived through it.

Then, a few weeks after that I heard a nice woman DJ and I started listening to her. We started talking back and forth and I really enjoyed talking with her. I tried to get her to come over to my apartment in Rockhill, but she would not because maybe again we were two women who were not lesbians. I have never been with a woman but I did do sexual things to her through my thought-broadcasting. I must admit that I enjoyed it. This went on for an extensive amount of time. I also listened to another person on the radio who told me that I was the second messiah. I thought to myself, *there is no second messiah, just Jesus Christ. Jesus Christ is the only, the one and only messiah who died for our sins, and showed us how to live a perfect life.* After a while I started saying that I am the second messiah, however, I know that there was no second messiah and it was not in the bible. I was thirty-three when my thought-broadcast came back. I told people that I was the second messiah. They tried to convince me that I was not and that nowhere in the bible did it mention that there were two messiahs. I also knew that the second messiah would not do sexual acts with someone of the opposite sex, let alone someone of the same sex! I had not lived an untarnished life and I have not, or had not lived to die on the cross for anyone's sins. Yet, I held on to this premise as long as I possibly could because it made me feel important. God is pure and lived a sin free life. He was sent here to be an example to all mankind. I feel that I am here to teach about hell, as I stated earlier in this book. I also was put here to show mankind that we are not supposed to think about sex without facing the repercussions. There did come a day when I didn't think about sex every chance I got alone. I'll get to this part later.

While I was communicating with this DJ the problem still went on with the nuisance neighbor so I decided to leave. I packed my things and had everything, except some necessities, put into storage. By then my schizophrenia was getting worse. All I did was think about suicide. I called the crisis center on a regular basis searching for intervention. I also called my mother talking suicide. The life intervention team and the poison intervention center could not promise that I would die. They, including my mother knew that I was trying to find a way to kill myself so they asked me why I wanted to know this. I didn't have any friends, I was not in contact with my other family members and I did not feel connected as far as employment. I did not have an address for the purposes of getting employment, and I had not handled, or God did not help me handle my thought-broadcast yet. It was hard to keep my thoughts clean, meaning sexually and suicide free. I reverted back to listening to gospel music and gospel shows. I really enjoyed listening to gospel music and talk because it freed me. However, I was still suicidal, and my money from my settlement was running out. It looked like I was headed back home. So after three months I moved back home with my parents. I was there for only two hours when I got a cab and went to Metropolitan Psych under the premise that I would be at the facility for about two weeks. Instead I was there for about a month and three weeks. I was quite disturbed that I had to stay so long. What got me committed for so long was that I had a plan and the fact that my momma testified to the fact that I was suicidal and had many plans. Another reason I had to stay was the nurses on my floor at the mental health facility put in my file that I was isolating and not participating in any of the life skills training groups. I just stayed in my room and didn't even want to leave the floor for breakfast, lunch and dinner. Then this nurse on my floor told me that the only way I was going to get released was if I went off the floor to different groups and I had to leave the floor for my meals; I complied. I think that the people at the facility took a liking to me when I showed that I could interact with them on a trusting level. I think they really were pulling for me and wanted me to handle my schizophrenia so that I could make it in the so-called normal society. I played volleyball, pool, basketball, cards, checkers, horse shoe and all the games at the carnival. It finally came to my release day and the only way they agreed to release me was because I showed them a photo album of me dressed appropriately and living in a clean apartment. I got a cab to my momma and dad's home. I had in my suitcase my clothes, my medicine and a referral to the Independence Center.

What is the Independence Center? The Independence Center is a mental health facility in St. Louis, MO that assists people with mental illness in integrating back into society. This means that they provide apartments, group homes, social security disability, SSI and food stamps. They also provide temporary employment, bus passes and lunches cooked by staff members. They also help members with getting Medicaid and call-a-ride. How this works is they provide members with a case worker who is in charge of helping with rides to their psychiatrist and other medical appointments. They also are in charge of helping members with anything and everything we need. However, the Independence Center comes later on in my life. They have helped me a lot!

After I left Metropolitan Psych I went back to my momma and dad's house. I took my radio with me. So later on that night I flipped to the station that the DJ that I had talked to for years was on and she was still there. I hung out with her from 7:00 P.M. to 12:00 midnight. After we talked a couple of days we were back to the sexual part of our relationship. I repeat this was only through my thought-broadcast abilities. It was not by any means in actuality. This was the perfect way of having sex and not getting STDs. I really did enjoy it back then. Again I isolated myself upstairs. I had months worth of medicine so I was feeling okay. The only thing was that I was not sleeping well, nor was I eating well. It was hot, and there was only a minimum amount of air coming out of the central air conditioner unit at my parents'. As time went on I grew more and more isolated. The only contact was whoever was on the radio. My DJ friend had gone to 10:00 A.M. to 2:00 P.M. There was a time when I went downstairs to use the bathroom. The phone rang and nobody responded. My nephew and I ended up in a fight. Afterward my niece and my nephew called my mother at work. After she got off work she told me that I had to leave. I told her that I would leave in the morning. I called the west end Independence Center and spoke with a man who worked there and he took me to a homeless shelter called Passage House. Passage House was a great place, even though there is no place like your own home. They provided three meals a day. We cleaned to get tickets for soap, toilet tissue and toothpaste. I like cleaning the women's and kids' bathroom. In the day after my chores, I went looking for a job. After I did this for a while, we all did life skills classes. I stayed here for approximately two months and then my social worker took me to Holtwood and introduced me to the Independence Center as a member. By this time the hallucinations were mostly auditory hallucinations and thought-broadcasting. By this time I believed that if you just thought of me you could hear me no matter how far away I was. I also still believed that I was the second messiah because if I was by someone who was sick I would feel it in my body. I remember this woman at Passage House was sick in front of me in the dinner line. I had to go to the end of the line and get away from her. While at Holtwood, this social worker's job was to take me to a food pantry because although we lived rent free we had to supply our own food. Well, I almost jumped out of his car because I felt so ill. It was like I was very, very weak. I was thinking when I was out of the sight of the sick person, I no longer felt as if I would pass out!

I informed my DJ friend that if she thought of me she could hear me during the times we were apart. She agreed that this was possible. At the end of my time at my momma's house and all of the time I was at the Passage House, I believed that all anyone had to do to hear me was to think about me. You know God can do anything; I believe this to be true. I know you are probably saying, "What else did she do besides hallucinate?" You cannot work when you are hallucinating. So again, take your medicine! Someone hallucinating would not know if someone were talking or not. An example would be if the schizophrenics hear, "you are fired." They may walk off their job because they think that someone fired them.

Thus far I still have dreams. I am working towards becoming an attorney. I have an associate degree as a paralegal, I have two other diplomas as a paralegal, a criminal justice diploma and a bookkeeping/accounting diploma. I have a certificate in paralegal studies from the American Bar Association, approved studies in legal studies and certification from Webster University. I have one hundred and ten credits towards my BA in legal studies at Webster University in St. Louis, MO. I have authored seven children's books as well as this book. I worked as an intern as a research paralegal. I worked for the housing court of the City of St. Louis. I worked for thirty-two different companies through the temporary services. I worked as a legal secretary for

CORE. I worked as an office assistant for a tax firm and, as an office assistant for Macy's Department Stores Company. I worked as a teacher-tutor of SLATE and for Walnut Park Community Church Organization. My first job was Six Flags over mid-America.

I consider myself as being well rounded, but sometimes I'm still hearing things even on my medicines. To break it down again I take thirteen psychiatric medicines. I take 7 10mg capsules of Loxapine; this adds up to be 1 70mg capsule. I also take 2 400mg tablets and 1 200 mg tablets of Seroquel. Both Loxapine and Seroquel are antipsychotics. I take an antidepressant called Citalopram in the amount of 1 40mg tablet. I also take 1 30mg tablet of Haldol; again this is an antipsychotic. Last, I take 1 1mg tablet called Benztropine. Benztropine is used for the purposes of alleviating side effects of all the psychiatric medicines.

Now, while I was at Holtwood there came a hallucination that I took to heart. I awoke and something was off. I heard a voice claiming to be Jesus Christ telling me that it was okay to curse. This voice was using a lot of profanity and I said, "This can't be Jesus." It also answered me when I asked, "Why did you take my family through this?"

The voice answered, "Because you all were always trying to do what was right." I got up and walked up and down Midland Ave. until I could not hear this voice anymore. I knew that it was a demon of schizophrenia because God does not use profanity to calm down his children. All he does is try to encourage us to be closer to him. I felt that God was trying to intervene when he said that we were always trying to do what was right. The devil or the demons of schizophrenia would not say anything encouraging like this. It really made me feel blessed. It states as do you believe him (Satan) or do you believe him, (Jesus Christ). By all means I chose Jesus' word.

Not too long from this day, I got into it with a female. So the next day I was taken to another group home called Rosati. I was very upset that I had to leave Holtwood. It was in a nice neighborhood in Overland, MO. Rosati was in a bad neighborhood where the majority of the buildings were vacant.

The bedroom that I was in was okay and of course I had my radio with me talking to this same DJ. I tried on several occasions to get her to come and get me and take me to a hotel. She never showed up. In retrospect I am glad that she didn't show up. However, I can admit that the fact that her not showing up was making me get bored with the radio relationship, if you can call it a relationship. This DJ woman and all the rest of the people I met was just a way to fulfill my time and my unrest as a person who could talk to the radio and TV.

This happening was just the way to increase my faith. I know real well that nobody but Jesus Christ could do this and I am sure that this is the perception of me. When people hear or see me they immediately think, *God did that!* I have seen people who have said, "How?" when I was listening to their radio or TV show.

While at Rosati I had an argument with one girl and one guy. Both times I was taken by ambulance with a police escort to Metropolitan Psychiatry. I stayed two weeks both times. While I was in the hospital I grew more and more paranoid because the close watch they kept on us made or exacerbated the situation. The fact that every door would lock behind and in front of me aggravated me to no end. After my two hospitalizations I was chosen to have my own apartment. I got the apartment and have been here for eighteen years.

Two years later my momma died from colon cancer. I am glad that I had my own place before she died; that way she didn't have to worry about me. She died a year after her diagnosis. She died because cancer spread throughout her body including her bones. In her last days she was in a lot of pain. Even though I knew that she had cancer, I never would have known that she had only seven days to live. I miss her a lot but due to my large family of four girls and three boys and my dad, she encouraged us to live on.

Not only did my momma encourage us to live on, but she also said before we knew that she had cancer that she didn't want any of us coming into her hospital room screaming and crying. She wanted us to handle her diagnosis like God has sent for her and that's how we acted. I felt so bad for my dad because he loved her like nobody could love her. He really placed his love for her and her love for him on a pedestal. They needed each other like no other couple did. She died at about 2:30 in the morning. When they let her come home they said that she had only five more days to live, but she lasted for seven. While I didn't go to see her for the last time because of the thought-broadcast, I was at home jumping and praying that she go into remission. I begged, pleaded and prayed that she stay alive. However, she didn't, so it must have been time for her to die. What kind of mother raises a person or child who could talk to the TV or radio? Well, my momma was strong and a good role model for me and my sisters and brothers. She was a strong disciplinarian. She said that we would put God first, and that serving the Lord would come first. She taught us not to curse or call each other out of our names. We could not fight each other, but if we were in a fight with someone outside of the family we had better help. We could not disrespect our elders or else we would get a whipping. She was an excellent cook. She could cook anything and it was good. My favorite foods of hers were dressing, greens, chitterlings and peach cobbler. She worked in a hospital called Connect Care, as a medical record supervisor. We all loved and needed her. She put us first, second and last on every occasion. She was very accepting of all people. Even in her pain, she was uplifting and inspiring. She taught us to put God first, and then family and then friends whom we were taught to treat just like family. I learned a lot from her about this world. She told me one day, "No matter what happens to you, you keep going." I was so proud that she saw me this way.

Maybe some of what I was going through helped her trust in Jesus in the midst of her storms. With my momma being dead at the young age of sixty-eight, my momma and dad had been together for fifty-four years, since they were fourteen years old. My dad who is eighty-three was also a good role model. He kept jobs and they were good jobs. He worked for ACF Industries as a burner's assistant, Footlockers and General Motors. He had several good jobs and has always taken good care of us. He was a good disciplinarian. All he had to do was look at us and we would start crying. There never was a time when he mistreated us. My momma and dad were both my heroes. At eighty-three he now has mild dementia, and I keep seeing little spurts of his true and happy self. I love both of them deeply. I can't wait to see my momma and tell her I wrote this book, and seven children's books.

A little about my brothers and sisters—they have all been in the workforce for forty years plus. This includes my oldest sister and my oldest brother. My next to oldest sister and brother worked for thirty-eight years. My twin brother has also worked for over thirty years. Last but not least, my baby sister has worked for over thirty years. I have three nieces, three nephews, four aunts, one uncle and a host of cousins, God sisters and God brothers. My great aunt is over one hundred and one years old.

My best friend who is sixty-two helped me get through my eighteen years at the apartment that I currently live in. We have known each other for about nineteen years. When I didn't have food to eat, she brought me some of hers. She helps me a lot through working, doing her chores and keeping food on the table.

After 2002, and the burial of my momma, I isolated and just withdrew deep into my darkest hour. I still talked to the DJ woman. I cried and cried. The only thing that kept me going was my two young nephews and my tiny little niece. I began to get better when my baby sister and her husband came to visit me often. I really enjoyed seeing them.

I must also say that my best friends and I both have schizophrenia and we met through the Independence Center. They encouraged me to befriend her.

Now I know that you are probably wondering if I was born this way or had it come into my life when I was younger. The answer is yes. I don't know how many of you have in your younger years watched *Romper Room*. Well I did every morning with my twin brother and baby sister. For those who watched recall that at the beginning or at the end of *Romper Room*, the host held a mirror up to her, gave and would say different people's names. She said, "And I see Ben, Dave, and Tony."

Well one day I was watching and I kept saying, "Shelley, Shelley, Shelley."

Then she said, "I see Shelley." I was smiling from ear to ear.

I said to my twin Sheldon, "She don't see you." That was fun but when I asked my momma if she could hear me she angrily said "no!" Even as a four-year-old child, I knew if one can hear me then so could others. So I went over to the radio. I don't recall what it was that I said, but I was talking to the radio. My momma saw me smiling back at the radio so she smiled at me and told whomever it was she was talking to on the telephone that I had a new friend. The woman on the radio smiled back at me.

Don't you want to know of the different ways other than suicide that I tried to get rid of the thought-broadcasting? Well first as I mentioned before I listened to gospel programs both on the TV and radio. Secondly I thought about sex a lot and my thinking was, *I am sure God does not want me thinking about sex with something he sent me, so maybe he would change me.* Third I was hypnotized twice. The first time I was hypnotized it was with a male and I thought, *this would be a perfect time and means to get rid of my thought-broadcasting.* The male hypnotized me and said that the next time someone was listening to my thoughts to say, "Roll the gates down," and this would block my thoughts.

The first time he said that I was not relaxed enough and that I would hinder the process if I did not relax. The second time I was hypnotized by a lady. She told me that I was the perfect person because I was very relaxed. I got home and each time it was the same; nothing had changed. The lady hypnotist explained my thought-broadcast as my subconscious mind taking over my conscious mind! I like this explanation!

Today I have not had the rapings and beatings for about fifteen years. I have not really engaged in sexual acts with anyone since 1997. I have really not thought about sex for about ten years.

I am proud to be chosen as a willing vessel of God's. Surely I could have lashed out and rebelled against God. In fact I did lash out, hence all the vivid sexual acts.

I hope that I have taken you all deep into what schizophrenia is! You all know now that schizophrenia is not just a white man's disease. It is very diverse. If you have a family member who exhibits any of these symptoms, get them help immediately! Don't think that it will simply go away. It won't go away, because there is no cure. We, schizophrenics, will always have to take medication.

Thank you for buying my book and I hope that I was fully clear enough that you understand what schizophrenia is about! God bless you! Keep the faith!